NATURAL ERECTILE DYSFUNCTION'S REMEDY

Unlocking the Power of Nature to Treat and Prevent Erectile Dysfunction, Enhance Mood, and Boost Energy and Stamina Levels for a Long-Lasting Erection with an Electrifying Orgasm

MRS. VERA JACOB

Copyright Notice. By Mrs. Vera Jacob

Table of Contents

INTRODUCTION

In the realm of human experience, there exists an intricate web of emotions, connections, and desires, with one particular aspect of our lives that has been cherished, celebrated, and cherished again throughout the ages, intimacy. The profound and beautiful act of coming together with a loved one, and forging a connection unlike any other, has been the source of joy and fulfillment for countless souls.

Yet, there are times when this intimate connection is marred by a silent, often stigmatized intruder called "Erectile Dysfunction (ED)". For those whom this intruder has visited and are suffering both physically and emotionally, that they have given up on their sex life, have lost their self-esteem, are scared of lovemaking, or suffering from any form and type of erectile dysfunction, fear not for salvation has come!

In this book titled "Natural Erectile Dysfunction's Remedy," the author will journey you through a step-by-step guide on discovery, empowerment, and transformation to battle against any form and type of erectile dysfunction (ED), boost your testosterone level, enhance mood, boost energy and stamina level, and help you to regain control of your sexual health and reignite the flames of passion in your life naturally without any side effect.

CHAPTER ONE
What Is Erectile Dysfunction?

Erectile dysfunction can be a sign of a physical or psychological condition. It can cause stress, relationship strain and low self-confidence.

The main symptom is a man's inability to get or keep an erection firm enough for sexual intercourse.

People suffering from any types or form of erectile dysfunction (ED) should in a matter of urgency, evaluated the ED to ascertain if it is caused by physical or psychological conditions and if the cause wasn't ascertained, or even if it was, don't be panic, the result is right now on your system or iPad or phones as "Natural Erectile Dysfunction's Remedy" got your back.

The Importance of Natural Remedies

The importance of natural remedies for managing and overcoming erectile dysfunction (ED) is a central theme in the book "Natural Erectile Dysfunction's Remedy." Here are some key points highlighting the significance of natural remedies:

1. Holistic Approach: Natural remedies encompass a holistic approach to addressing ED. Unlike some pharmaceutical options that target only the physical symptoms, natural remedies consider the interconnectedness of physical, emotional, and psychological factors. This approach aims to treat the root causes of ED rather than just the symptoms.

2. Minimal Side Effects: Many pharmaceutical ED medications can come with unwanted side effects, ranging from headaches to digestive issues. Natural

remedies, when used correctly, are often gentler on the body and have fewer adverse effects, making them a preferred choice for those seeking a more natural and balanced solution.

3. Long-Term Health Benefits: Natural remedies not only address ED but can also have a positive impact on overall health. For example, adopting a healthier diet and lifestyle choices can lead to benefits beyond improved sexual function, such as better cardiovascular health, reduced risk of chronic diseases, and increased vitality.

4. Empowerment: The use of natural remedies empowers individuals to take an active role in their health and well-being. By making informed choices about nutrition, exercise, and lifestyle, individuals can regain a sense of control over their bodies and

their ED, promoting a sense of self-efficacy and confidence.

5. Reduced Dependency: Relying on pharmaceuticals for ED can sometimes lead to dependency and a psychological reliance on the medication. Natural remedies can provide a path to reducing or eliminating the need for medication over time, allowing for greater independence and self-sufficiency.

6. Customization: Natural remedies offer a wide range of options, allowing individuals to customize their approach based on their specific needs and preferences. What works for one person may not work for another, and natural remedies provide the flexibility to tailor solutions to individual circumstances.

7. Long-Term Sustainability: The sustainability of natural remedies is a key consideration. Rather than relying on a finite supply of medication, natural approaches often involve sustainable lifestyle changes that can be maintained over the long term, promoting ongoing sexual health and well-being.

8. Respect for Nature: Natural remedies often respect and harness the wisdom of nature. Many herbs, supplements, and dietary strategies have been used for centuries in various traditional healing systems. This approach aligns with the idea of working in harmony with the natural world to achieve wellness.

In "Natural Erectile Dysfunction's Remedy," these aspects of natural remedies are explored, providing readers with a comprehensive understanding of how they can take control of their sexual health and overall well-being. By emphasizing the importance of natural solutions, the book empowers individuals to make informed choices that can lead to lasting improvements in their lives, fostering hope and optimism in the face of ED.

The Causes and Risk Factors

Erectile Dysfunction (ED) is a complex condition with a myriad of potential causes and risk factors. Understanding these underlying factors is the first step towards finding an effective natural remedy. In this chapter, we'll delve into the multifaceted world of ED, exploring its origins and the various elements that contribute to its development.

Physical Causes of Erectile Dysfunction

Erectile Dysfunction (ED) can have various physical causes that interfere with the normal physiological processes required for achieving and maintaining an erection. Some common causes of erectile dysfunction (ED) that are physical include:

1. Vascular Issues: Problems with blood flow are a leading physical cause of ED. Conditions that affect the blood vessels can impede the proper flow of blood to the penis. Atherosclerosis, a condition characterized by the buildup of fatty plaques in the arteries, can restrict blood flow and lead to ED.

2. Hormonal Imbalances: Hormones play a crucial role in regulating sexual function. Having low amount of testosterone level which is the primary male sex hormone, can lead to ED. Hormonal imbalances may result from conditions like hypogonadism or certain medical treatments.

3. Nerve Damage: Nerves play a key role in transmitting

signals from the brain to the penis to initiate and maintain an erection. Nerve damage can occur due to various factors, including injuries, surgery (such as prostate surgery), or medical conditions like diabetes. Diabetic neuropathy, for example, can affect nerve function and lead to ED.

4. Medications and Medical Conditions: Certain medications and underlying medical conditions can interfere with the ability to achieve and sustain an erection. Medications like some antihypertensives, antidepressants, and antipsychotics can have ED as a side effect. Medical conditions such as multiple sclerosis, Parkinson's disease, and Peyronie's disease can also contribute to ED.

5. Penile Anomalies: Physical abnormalities or structural issues in the penis can lead to ED.

Conditions like Peyronie's disease, which involves the development of scar tissue in the penis, can cause bending or curvature that makes erections painful or difficult.

6. Injury or Trauma: Past injuries or trauma to the pelvic area, spinal cord, or genitals can result in physical damage that affects the mechanisms involved in achieving an erection.

7. Prostate Issues: The prostate gland and its surrounding structures are critical for the proper functioning of the male reproductive system. Conditions like an enlarged prostate (benign prostatic hyperplasia) or prostate cancer and their treatments can impact erectile function.

8. Smoking and Substance Abuse: Smoking and the use of substances such as recreational drugs or excessive

alcohol can contribute to vascular issues, which, in turn, can lead to ED.

9. Obesity and Poor Diet: Being overweight or obese is associated with an increased risk of ED. Poor dietary choices and a lack of physical activity can contribute to obesity and negatively impact vascular health.

Understanding the physical causes of ED is essential for both individuals experiencing ED and healthcare professionals. Identifying the specific cause or contributing factors can guide the development of an appropriate treatment plan, including natural remedies, lifestyle changes, or medical interventions, to address the underlying physical issues and improve erectile function.

Psychological Causes of Erectile Dysfunction

Psychological factors can play a significant role in the

development of Erectile Dysfunction (ED). These factors can affect the brain's ability to send the necessary signals to initiate and maintain an erection. Some basic causes of erectile dysfunction that is caused psychologically are:

1. Stress and Anxiety: Stress, whether related to work, finances, relationships, or other life events, can lead to elevated levels of the stress hormone cortisol. Anxiety about sexual performance or other life stressors can create a "fight or flight" response in the body, which can interfere with the relaxation of blood vessels and muscle tissues necessary for an erection.

2. Depression: Depression is a mood disorder that can affect various aspects of a person's life, including sexual function. The persistent feeling of sadness, hopelessness, and lack of interest in activities can reduce libido and inhibit the brain's ability to respond

to sexual stimuli.

3. Performance Anxiety: Worries about sexual performance, especially if they have been associated with previous instances of ED, can create a self-perpetuating cycle. The fear of not being able to perform sexually can lead to ED, which then reinforces performance anxiety.

4. Relationship Issues: Problems in a romantic relationship, such as communication difficulties, unresolved conflicts, or emotional distance, can contribute to ED. A lack of emotional intimacy can affect a person's ability to become sexually aroused and maintain an erection.

5. Body Image Concerns: Negative body image or low self-esteem can affect sexual confidence and contribute to ED. These issues may be related to

unrealistic expectations about one's own appearance or a perceived lack of attractiveness.

6. Sexual Trauma or Past Experiences: Past traumatic experiences, including sexual abuse or assault, can have a lasting impact on a person's mental and emotional well-being, potentially leading to sexual difficulties, including ED.

7. Guilt or Shame: Feelings of guilt or shame related to sexuality, religious or cultural beliefs, or previous sexual experiences can interfere with the ability to engage in and enjoy sexual activity.

8. Lack of Desire: A lack of sexual desire or interest in sexual activity, known as hypoactive sexual desire disorder, can be psychological in nature and lead to ED. This may be related to relationship issues, stress, or other emotional factors.

It's important to note that psychological factors can often interact with physical causes of ED. For example, a man with physical issues, such as vascular problems, may develop performance anxiety related to his ED, compounding the problem. Additionally, stress, anxiety, and depression can also have physical effects on the body, such as impacting blood flow and hormone levels.

Addressing the psychological causes of ED often involves a combination of therapies, including counseling or therapy to address emotional and relationship issues, stress reduction techniques, and mindfulness practices. Open communication with a healthcare provider or therapist is essential to identify and manage these psychological factors effectively and find the right approach to overcome ED.

Lifestyle and Environmental Risk Factors

Erectile Dysfunction (ED) is a multifaceted condition influenced not only by physical and psychological factors but also by various lifestyle and environmental elements. This chapter delves into the lifestyle choices we make and the external factors we encounter that can contribute to ED. Recognizing and addressing these risk factors is crucial in the quest for natural remedies and the restoration of sexual health.

1. Smoking and substance and abuse: these are lifestyle choices that can significantly contribute to the development and exacerbation of Erectile Dysfunction (ED).

2. Recreational Drugs and Alcohol: Recreational drugs and excessive alcohol consumption can significantly contribute to the development and worsening of

Erectile Dysfunction (ED). This section delves into the effects of recreational drugs and alcohol on sexual function and ED, emphasizing the importance of understanding these factors in the pursuit of natural remedies for ED.

3. Obesity and Poor Diet: In the journey towards a natural remedy for Erectile Dysfunction (ED), it's essential to address lifestyle factors, and among these, as obesity and dietary choices play a significant role.

4. Other Lifestyle Considerations like, tight clothing, hot baths, and saunas can affect testicular temperature and potentially contribute to ED.

5. Understanding the role of lifestyle and environmental risk factors in the development of ED is paramount. By making informed choices, adopting healthier

lifestyles, and minimizing exposure to harmful environmental influences, individuals can significantly reduce the risk of ED. This chapter provides a foundation for embracing natural remedies and lifestyle changes to regain control over sexual health and overall well-being.

CHAPTER TWO
The Role of Nutrition

Proper nutrition is a cornerstone of a holistic approach to remedying Erectile Dysfunction (ED) naturally. This chapter delves into the crucial role that nutrition plays in improving sexual health and enhancing erectile function. By understanding the impact of dietary choices and nutrients, individuals can take significant steps toward overcoming ED and regaining control of their sexual well-being.

Dietary Choices and Their Impact

The choices we make in our diets have a profound impact on our overall health and, importantly, on our sexual well-being. This section explores the connection between dietary choices and their influence on Erectile Dysfunction (ED). Understanding how specific foods and dietary patterns affect sexual health is a pivotal step in the journey toward a natural remedy for ED.

Nutrition plays a vital role in sexual health and can significantly impact erectile function. This subsection explores key nutrients, vitamins, minerals, and macronutrients that are essential for promoting healthy erectile function. By incorporating these nutrient-rich foods into your diet, you can support your sexual vitality and work toward a natural remedy for Erectile Dysfunction (ED).

Foods that can help alleviate ED

Nutrient-Rich Foods for Erectile Health include and not limited to:

1. L-Arginine: This amino acid is a precursor to nitric oxide, a molecule that plays a crucial role in relaxing blood vessels and promoting blood flow to the penis.

Foods rich in L-arginine include nuts, seeds, and lean proteins like chicken and turkey.

2. Zinc: Zinc is essential for the production of testosterone, a hormone vital for sexual function. Incorporate zinc-rich foods like oysters, lean meats, beans, and nuts into your diet.

3. Folate (Vitamin B9): Folate is necessary for overall sexual health and may help improve sperm quality. Greens, citrus fruits, and legumes are superb sources of folate.

4. Vitamin D: Vitamin D is associated with testosterone production and may help enhance erectile function. Get your daily dose of vitamin D from sunlight, fatty fish like salmon, fortified dairy products, and supplements if necessary.

5. Omega-3 Fatty Acids: These healthy fats can improve

blood flow and arterial health. Fatty fish (salmon, mackerel), flaxseeds, chia seeds, and walnuts are rich sources of omega-3 fatty acids.

6. Antioxidants: Antioxidants combat oxidative stress and inflammation, which can impair vascular function and lead to ED. Foods like berries, dark chocolate, and fruits high in vitamin C, such as oranges and strawberries, are packed with antioxidants.

7. Nitrates: Nitrates are transformed into nitric oxide in the body system that helps to relax blood vessels. Nitrate-rich foods include beets, spinach, and arugula.

8. Magnesium: Magnesium contributes to vascular health and may help with blood flow. dark chocolate, spinach and almonds are excellent sources of

magnesium.

9. Watermelon: Watermelon contains an amino acid called citrulline, which can have a similar effect to L-arginine in promoting nitric oxide production.

Incorporating these nutrient-rich foods into your diet can provide a solid foundation for enhancing erectile health. A balanced diet that prioritizes these nutrients can contribute to improved sexual function and overall well-being.

Creating a Balanced Diet Plan

Creating a balanced diet plan that prioritizes sexual health and overall well-being is essential in the journey to finding a natural remedy for Erectile Dysfunction (ED). This subsection provides practical guidance on crafting a well-rounded diet that incorporates nutrient-rich foods and essential dietary principles to support erectile function.

These mixed include but not limited to:

1. Diversify Your Plate: Consume a variety of foods from different food groups, including fruits, vegetables, lean proteins, whole grains, and healthy fats. This ensures a broad spectrum of nutrients that promote sexual vitality.

2. Prioritize Whole Foods: opt for whole, unprocessed foods over highly processed options. Whole foods are rich in essential nutrients and free from additives that can negatively impact health.

3. Lean Proteins: Include lean sources of protein like poultry, fish, lean cuts of meat, tofu, and legumes. Protein is essential for tissue repair and hormone production, which are critical for sexual health.

4. Complex Carbohydrates: Choose complex carbohydrates like whole grains, legumes, and

starchy vegetables. These provide a steady source of energy and maintain blood sugar levels, important for overall well-being.

5. Portion Control: Be mindful of portion sizes to prevent overeating, which can lead to weight gain and obesity, both risk factors for ED.

6. Hydration: water is very essential for the body. However, it is very important that one stay sufficiently hydrated by drinking enough water. Proper hydration is vital for overall health and can improve sexual function.

7. Limit Added Sugars and Processed Foods: Minimize consumption of foods and beverages high in added sugars, as they can contribute to inflammation and poor blood sugar control.

A balanced diet that incorporates these principles not only

supports erectile function but also promotes overall health and vitality. By making informed dietary choices and adhering to a balanced diet plan, individuals can take a proactive role in improving their sexual health and well-being.

CHAPTER THREE
Herbal Remedies

Herbal remedies have been used for centuries to address various health concerns, including Erectile Dysfunction (ED). This chapter explores the world of herbal treatments and their potential role in a natural remedy for ED. Understanding the herbs that have shown promise in improving erectile function empowers individuals to explore alternative approaches to sexual health.

Herbs and Supplements

Herbal remedies have long been utilized to address a variety of health concerns, including Erectile Dysfunction (ED). This section explores some of the popular herbal remedies that have shown promise in improving erectile function and overall sexual health. Understanding these herbs empowers individuals to consider alternative approaches to ED management.

What Are the Herbs to Treat and Prevent Erectile Dysfunction?

The herbs to treat erectile dysfunctions include:

1. Panax Ginseng

2. Horny goat weed

3. Maca root

4. Yohimbine

5. Ginko Biloba

All You Need to About Panax Ginseng

Panax ginseng, commonly known as Asian or Korean ginseng, is a perennial plant belonging to the Araliaceae family. The word "Panax" is derived from the Greek word "panacea," which means "all-healing" or "universal remedy." Ginseng has been used for centuries in traditional Chinese medicine and is highly regarded for its adaptogenic properties.

Below are the properties of Panax Ginseng:

1. Adaptogenic Properties: Ginseng is classified as an adaptogen, meaning it is believed to help the body adapt to stress and maintain balance. It is thought to enhance the body's overall resilience and ability to cope with various stressors, whether physical, chemical, or biological.

2. Active Compounds: The primary active compounds in Panax ginseng are ginsenosides. These are the most essential compounds that contribute effectively for

the treatment of ED. The composition of ginsenosides can vary depending on factors such as the plant's age and how it is processed.

3. Traditional Uses: In traditional medicine, Panax ginseng has been used to address a variety of health concerns. It is often associated with improvements in energy, cognitive function, and overall vitality. It has also been used to support the immune system and promote general well-being.

4. Mental reasoning also known as cognitive reasoning: Some studies proved that Panax ginseng has the properties with the potential to enhance cognitive-enhancing effects. It is believed to potentially improve memory, concentration, and overall mental performance.

5. Energy and Stamina: Ginseng is commonly

associated with increased energy levels and improved stamina. It is sometimes used by individuals seeking a natural remedy for fatigue and a boost in physical performance.

6. Immune Support: Traditional uses and some research indicate that Panax ginseng may have immune-modulating effects, potentially supporting the immune system's function.

How to Prepare and Administer Panax Ginseng?

Panax ginseng is available in various forms, including fresh roots, dried roots, powders, capsules, and extracts. The method of preparation and administration can depend on the specific form of ginseng you have. Here are some general guidelines:

1. Fresh or Dried Roots: Chewing or Brewing Tea: You

can chew on a small piece of fresh or dried ginseng root. Alternatively, you can simmer the root in water to make ginseng tea. Simply steep the root in hot water for 15-20 minutes, then strain and drink.

2. Powder: Capsules or Tablets: Ginseng is commonly available in pre-measured capsules or tablets. Follow the recommended dosage on the product's label, and take it with water. This is a convenient way to ensure a standardized dose.

3. Extracts: Liquid Extracts: Ginseng extracts are often available in liquid form. Follow the dosage instructions on the product label, and mix the recommended amount with water or another beverage before consumption.

4. Dosage: Dosages can vary based on factors such as the individual's health, the specific product, and the

reason for use. It's crucial to follow the recommended dosage on the product's label or consult with a healthcare professional for personalized advice.

5. Timing: It is advisable that you consume this herb in the morning to help improved your energy levels. However, individual responses can vary, and some people may prefer taking it at different times of the day.

6. Cycle of Use: Some experts recommend cycling the use of ginseng, meaning taking it for a specific period and then taking a break. For example, you might use it for a few weeks or months and then take a break of a similar duration.

All you Need to Know About Horny Goat Weed

"Horny goat weed" is a common name for a flowering plant

known by its scientific name, Epimedium. The plant is native to Asia and the Mediterranean region and has been used in traditional Chinese medicine for centuries. The name "horny goat weed" is derived from the observation that goats and other animals seemed to become more sexually active after consuming the plant.

Here are key points about horny goat weed (Epimedium):

1. Traditional Use: In traditional Chinese medicine, Epimedium has been used to address various health concerns, including those related to sexual function. It is often promoted as an aphrodisiac and is believed to have potential benefits for libido and erectile function.

2. Active Compounds: Horny goat weed contains several bioactive compounds, including icariin, which is often considered the primary active

ingredient. Icariin is believed to have potential effects on the nitric oxide pathway, which plays a role in blood vessel dilation and erectile function.

3. Potential Benefits: Some studies and anecdotal evidence suggest that horny goat weed may have potential benefits for sexual health, including increased libido and improved erectile function. However, research on its effectiveness is still limited, and more studies are needed to confirm these potential benefits.

4. Forms of Administration: Horny goat weed is available in various forms, including capsules, powders, and extracts. The dosage and form of administration can vary based on the specific product, and it's essential to follow the recommended guidelines.

5. Caution and Side Effects: While horny goat weed is generally considered safe for many people when used in moderation, it can cause side effects in some individuals. These may include dizziness, rapid heart rate, and nausea. Individuals with pre-existing health conditions or those taking medications should consult with a healthcare professional before using horny goat weed.

6. Quality and Source: As with any herbal supplement, it's crucial to choose products from reputable sources to ensure quality and purity. The concentration of active ingredients can vary between different products.

How to Prepare and Administer Horny Goat

Weed?

To prepare and administer horny goat weed, it is important to know the various forms that we can have access to and how we can use it. Horny goat weed is available in various forms, and the method of preparation and administration can depend on the specific product you have. Here are some general guidelines:

1. Capsules or Tablets: This is one of the most common forms of administration. Follow the recommended dosage on the product's label, usually with water or a meal. Capsules provide a convenient and pre-measured way to take horny goat weed.

2. Powder: Some people prefer to use horny goat weed in powdered form. You can mix the recommended amount of powder with water, juice, or a smoothie. Make sure to follow the dosage instructions on the

product label.

3. Liquid Extract: Horny goat weed is also available in liquid extract form. Measure the recommended amount, usually using a dropper, and mix it with water or another beverage before consumption.

4. Dosage: Some individuals prepare horny goat weed as a tea. You can steep the dried herb in hot water for about 10-15 minutes, then strain and drink. for me, 15 minutes is the best option but you can adjust to your preferred time based on your capabilities and health level. Dosage: Dosages can vary based on factors such as the specific product, the concentration of active ingredients, and the individual's health. It's crucial to follow the recommended dosage on the product's label or consult with a healthcare professional for personalized advice.

5. Timing: The timing of administration can vary based on individual preferences and the specific product. Some people prefer taking it with meals, while others may take it at a specific time of day based on their routine.

6. Cycle of Use: Similar to other herbal supplements, some individuals choose to cycle the use of horny goat weed. This involves using it for a specific period and then taking a break. Consult with a healthcare professional for guidance on the appropriate cycle for your situation.

7. Caution and Consultation: Before incorporating horny goat weed into your routine, especially in larger or more concentrated forms, it's advisable to consult with a healthcare professional. This is particularly important if you have pre-existing health

conditions, take medications, or are pregnant.

All you Need to Know About Maca Root!

Maca root, scientifically known as Lepidium meyenii, it is a plant that belongs to the cruciferous vegetable family. It is native to the high-altitude regions of the Andes Mountains in Peru and has been cultivated and used as a food source for thousands of years. Maca is well-known for its edible root, which is often used for its potential health benefits and as a natural remedy. Here are some key benefits of the consumption of maca root:

1. Nutrient Content: Maca root is rich in several essential nutrients, including vitamins (such as B vitamins), minerals (including calcium and potassium), and fiber. It also contains bioactive compounds like glucosinolates and macaenes.

2. Adaptogenic Properties: Maca is often classified as an adaptogen, a substance believed to help the body adapt to various stressors, both physical and mental. It is thought to have the potential to enhance resilience and balance in the body.

3. Traditional Use: In traditional Peruvian medicine, maca has been used for various purposes, including improving energy, stamina, and fertility. It has also been traditionally used to address hormonal imbalances and support reproductive health.

4. Potential Benefits: While more research is needed to establish the full range of benefits, some studies and anecdotal evidence suggest that maca may have potential benefits, such as improved energy levels, enhanced libido, and support for hormonal balance.

How to Prepare and Administer Maca Root?

Maca root is available in various forms which include:

1. Powder: Often used in smoothies, beverages, or added to food.

2. Capsules or Tablets: Convenient for those who prefer a measured dosage.

3. Liquid Extracts: Concentrated forms of maca for those who may prefer this option.

4. Dosage: Dosages can vary based on factors such as the specific form of maca and individual health conditions. It's important to follow the recommended dosage on the product's label or consult with a healthcare professional.

5. Caution and Side Effects: While maca is generally considered safe for many people, it's essential to be aware of potential side effects and interactions. Some

individuals may experience digestive issues or hormonal changes. People with thyroid conditions should exercise caution due to compounds in maca that may affect thyroid function.

All You Need to Know About Yohimbine?

Yohimbine is an alkaloid derived from the bark of the Pausinystalia yohimbe tree, which is native to central and western Africa. It is also found in the bark of the related plant, Rauwolfia serpentina. Yohimbine has been used for various purposes, and its primary pharmacological effects are related to its action as an alpha-2 adrenergic receptor antagonist.

Here are key points about yohimbine:

1. Mechanism of Action: Yohimbine primarily acts as an antagonist of alpha-2 adrenergic receptors. These

receptors are involved in the regulation of neurotransmitters, including norepinephrine. By blocking alpha-2 receptors, yohimbine can increase the release of norepinephrine and other neurotransmitters, leading to various physiological effects.

2. Traditional Uses: Yohimbe bark has been used in traditional African medicine for various purposes, including as an aphrodisiac and to address issues related to sexual function. Yohimbine, as an isolated compound, has been studied for its potential effects on erectile dysfunction and sexual arousal.

3. Erectile Dysfunction: Yohimbine has been investigated for its potential use in treating erectile dysfunction. Some studies suggest that it may have a modest effect in improving erectile function, possibly

by increasing blood flow to the genital area.

4. Weight Loss: Yohimbine has also been studied for its potential role in weight loss. It is believed to enhance fat mobilization by increasing the release of fatty acids from adipose tissue.

5. Adverse Effects: Yohimbine can cause side effects, including increased heart rate, elevated blood pressure, anxiety, and gastrointestinal discomfort. These effects can be more pronounced at higher doses. Individuals with cardiovascular issues, anxiety disorders, or certain medical conditions may be more sensitive to these effects.

6. Interactions: Yohimbine may interact with certain medications, particularly those affecting blood pressure and heart function. It's important to inform your healthcare provider about any supplements or

medications you are taking.

7. Regulation: Yohimbine is available as a dietary supplement in some countries, but it is regulated, and its sale may be restricted in others. Always choose reputable sources when considering yohimbine supplements.

How to Prepare and Administer Yohmibine?

Yohimbine is commonly available in supplement form, typically as capsules or liquid extracts. It's important to follow the recommended dosage instructions on the product's label, and if in doubt, consult with a healthcare professional for personalized guidance. Here are general guidelines for preparing and administering yohimbine supplements:

1. Capsules: the dosage: please follow the dosage

recommended on the label of the product you have/purchase. Remember that capsules usually provide a pre-measured dose of yohimbine.

2. Administration: Take the capsules with a full glass of water, and it's often advisable to take them with a meal to minimize the risk of stomach upset.

3. Liquid Extract: Dosage: Measure the recommended amount using the dropper provided with the product or another measuring tool.

4. Mixing with Beverages: Yohimbine liquid extract can be mixed with water or another beverage to make it more palatable. Follow the dosage instructions, and ensure that you mix it thoroughly before consumption.

5. Timing: Yohimbine is often taken on an empty stomach or with a small meal. However, individual

responses can vary, so it's advisable to follow the specific recommendations provided with the product or consult with a healthcare professional.

6. Cycle of Use: Some individuals may choose to cycle the use of yohimbine, meaning they use it for a specific period and then take a break. This can help minimize the potential for tolerance and reduce the risk of side effects over time. If considering a cycling approach, it's important to consult with a healthcare professional.

7. Caution and Monitoring: Yohimbine can have stimulant-like effects, so it's essential to monitor your response and be aware of potential side effects. Pay attention to changes in heart rate, blood pressure, and any signs of anxiety or gastrointestinal discomfort.

If you experience any adverse effects or have

concerns about its use, consult with a healthcare professional promptly.

8. Interactions: Be aware of potential interactions with medications, particularly those affecting blood pressure and heart function. Inform your healthcare provider about any supplements or medications you are taking to ensure there are no contraindications.

All You Need to Know About Ginko Biloba?

Ginkgo, or Ginkgo biloba, is one of the oldest living tree species and is often referred to as a "living fossil." The tree is native to China and has distinctive fan-shaped leaves. Ginkgo has a long history of use in traditional Chinese medicine, and its leaves are commonly used to prepare herbal extracts for medicinal purposes.

Here are key points about ginkgo:

1. Active Compounds: Ginkgo leaves contain a variety of bioactive compounds, including flavonoids and terpenoids which are believed to be the medicinal properties of the plant's.

2. Traditional Uses: Ginkgo has been used in traditional medicine for centuries. In traditional Chinese medicine, it has been employed to address various health concerns, including respiratory and circulatory issues.

3. Cognitive Function: Ginkgo has gained popularity in modern times for its potential cognitive benefits. Some studies suggest that ginkgo extract may have neuroprotective effects and could potentially improve memory and cognitive function, particularly in individuals with age-related cognitive decline.

4. Peripheral Circulation: Ginkgo is known for its

potential to improve blood circulation, particularly in the peripheral arteries. This has led to its use in addressing conditions such as intermittent claudication (painful walking due to reduced blood flow) and tinnitus (ringing in the ears).

5. Antioxidant Properties: Ginkgo has antioxidant properties, which means it may help neutralize harmful free radicals in the body. This antioxidant activity is thought to contribute to its potential protective effects on cells and tissues.

6. Caution and Side Effects: While ginkgo is generally considered safe for many people, it can cause side effects in some individuals. Such as: gastrointestinal discomfort, headache, and dizziness. Ginkgo may also interact with certain medications, so it's crucial to consult with a healthcare professional, especially if

you are taking blood-thinning medications.

7. Quality and Source: Choose ginkgo supplements from reputable sources to ensure product quality and purity. Look for standardized extracts and products that have undergone third-party testing.

How to Prepare and Administer Ginko Biloba?

Ginkgo biloba is commonly available in various forms, including capsules, tablets, liquid extracts, and dried leaves for tea. The method of preparation and administration can depend on the specific product you have. Here are general guidelines:

1. Capsules or Tablets: the dosage: please follow the dosage recommended on the label of the product you

have/purchase. Capsules and tablets typically provide a pre-measured dose of ginkgo biloba.

2. Administration: Take the capsules or tablets with a full glass of water, preferably with a meal.

3. Liquid Extract: Dosage: Measure the recommended amount using the dropper provided with the product or another measuring tool.

4. Mixing with Beverages: Ginkgo biloba liquid extract can be mixed with water or another beverage to make it more palatable. Follow the dosage instructions, and ensure that you mix it thoroughly before consumption.

5. Tea: Dried Leaves: Some people prefer to make ginkgo biloba tea using dried leaves. Steep one teaspoon of dried ginkgo biloba leaves in hot water for about 10-15 minutes. Strain and drink.

6. Timing: Ginkgo biloba is often taken with meals to enhance absorption and minimize the risk of stomach upset. However, individual responses can vary, so it's advisable to follow the specific recommendations provided with the product or consult with a healthcare professional.

All You Need to Know about L-argine?

L-arginine is a building block protein known as an amino acid. It is classified as a semi-essential or conditionally essential amino acid, meaning that while the body can typically produce it, there are situations where the body may not produce enough, and supplementation becomes necessary.

Here are key points about L-arginine:

1. Biological Functions: L-arginine plays a crucial role in various physiological processes. It is the originator of nitric oxide (NO), a molecule that helps dilate and relax the blood vessels. This vasodilatory effect is important for maintaining healthy blood flow and cardiovascular function.

2. Nitric Oxide Production: The conversion of L-arginine to nitric oxide is carried out by enzymes called nitric oxide synthases (NOS). Nitric oxide has vasodilatory effects, contributing to the regulation of blood pressure and blood flow.

3. Sources: L-arginine is naturally found in protein-rich foods, including red meat, poultry, fish, dairy products, and certain plant sources like nuts and seeds. Additionally, the body can synthesize L-arginine from other amino acids.

4. Supplementation: L-arginine is available as a dietary supplement, and it's often promoted for various health purposes. Some people use L-arginine supplements to support cardiovascular health, improve exercise performance, or enhance recovery.

5. Exercise Performance: There is some research suggesting that L-arginine supplementation may have potential benefits for exercise performance, particularly in situations where blood flow and oxygen delivery to muscles are critical.

6. Cardiovascular Health: L-arginine has been studied for its potential cardiovascular benefits, including its role in supporting healthy blood pressure and improving endothelial function (the function of the inner lining of blood vessels).

7. Wound Healing: L-arginine is involved in the synthesis of proteins and collagen, making it important for wound healing and tissue repair.

8. Caution and Interactions: While L-arginine is generally considered safe for most people, it may interact with certain medications, such as those for blood pressure or erectile dysfunction. Individuals with certain health conditions, including herpes infections, should use L-arginine with caution.

How to Prepare and Administer L-arginine

L-arginine is commonly available as a dietary supplement in various forms, including capsules, tablets, powders, and liquid formulations. The method of preparation and administration can depend on the specific product you have. Here are general guidelines:

1. Capsules or Tablets: the dosage: please follow the dosage recommended on the label of the product you have/purchase. Capsules and tablets typically provide a pre-measured dose of L-arginine.

2. Administration: Take the capsules or tablets with a full glass of water, preferably between meals or as directed on the product label.

3. Powder: Dosage: Measure the recommended amount of L-arginine powder using a scoop or other measuring tool.

4. Mixing with Beverages: L-arginine powder can be mixed with water, juice, or a smoothie to make it more palatable. Ensure that you mix it thoroughly before consumption.

5. Liquid Formulation: Dosage: Measure the recommended amount of liquid L-arginine using a dropper or other measuring tool.

6. Mixing with Beverages: Liquid L-arginine can be mixed with water or another beverage for easier consumption.

7. Timing: L-arginine is often recommended to be taken on an empty stomach or between meals to enhance absorption. However, individual responses can vary, and it's advisable to follow the specific recommendations provided with the product or consult with a healthcare professional.

CHAPTER FOUR
Lifestyle Changes
The Importance of Exercise

Regular physical activity can improve blood circulation, cardiovascular health, and over-all well-being. Take part in aerobic exercises such as; jogging, walking, cycling, and swimming and Incorporate strength training exercises to boost testosterone levels and improve muscle mass. Maintain a healthy weight, as obesity is a risk factor for ED. Regulating your meal and the consumption of a balanced diet meal plus regular exercise have the potency to maintain a healthy weight.

Managing Stress and Anxiety

Managing stress and anxiety is crucial for improving erectile dysfunction (ED) of psychological origin. Here are some strategies to help with stress and anxiety related to natural erectile dysfunction:

Be honest and open to your partner: communication with your partner in an honest manner is essential step to taking charge of your sex life. Discuss your concerns and feelings, and ensure they are supportive and understanding. Mutual understanding can help reduce anxiety.

Practice relaxation techniques: Taking slow, deep breaths can help calm your nervous system and reduce anxiety.

Progressive muscle relaxation: This involves tensing and then relaxing each muscle group to relieve physical tension.

Mindfulness and meditation: Mindfulness techniques can help you stay present and reduce stress and anxiety.

Regular exercise: Physical activity can reduce stress and anxiety, improve blood flow, and enhance overall health. Make sure you undergo at least 150 minutes of a regular intensity exercise every week.

Healthy diet: Eating a balanced diet rich in fruits, vegetables, whole grains, lean proteins, and healthy fats can improve overall health and support better sexual function.

Get enough sleep: Quality sleep is essential for stress management and overall well-being. Ensure you have at least 7-9 hours' sleep every night.

Manage your stressors: Identify and address the sources of your stress and anxiety. This may involve time management, setting realistic goals, or seeking professional help if necessary.

Limit alcohol and caffeine: Excessive consumption of alcohol and caffeine can contribute to anxiety and affect sexual performance. Moderation is key.

Seek professional help: If your stress and anxiety are

severely impacting your life and ED, consider speaking with a therapist, counselor, or psychiatrist. Cognitive-behavioral therapy (CBT) is often effective in managing ED related to psychological factors.

Medication options: In some cases, your healthcare provider may recommend medications to help manage your anxiety or ED. You can combine these with other strategies.

Lifestyle changes: Address other lifestyle factors that can contribute to ED, such as smoking, excessive drinking, or drug use. Quitting smoking and reducing alcohol or drug use can have a positive impact on your sexual function.

Supplements and herbs: Some natural supplements, such as L-arginine, ginseng, and maca root, have been studied for their potential benefits in improving erectile function. However, consult with a healthcare professional before using any supplements.

Stay patient and positive: It's important to remember that stress and anxiety-related ED can be temporary, and improvement may take time. Maintaining a positive attitude and staying patient can be helpful.

Always consult a healthcare professional for personalized advice on managing ED and any underlying psychological issues. They can help you determine the most appropriate treatment plan tailored to your specific needs.

Sleep and Erectile Health

Sleep plays a significant role in maintaining overall health, and it can also impact erectile health. Poor sleep quality and insufficient sleep can contribute to erectile dysfunction (ED) and other sexual health issues. Here's how sleep and erectile health are interconnected:

Hormone regulation: Sleep is essential for the regulation of hormones, including testosterone. Testosterone is a key hormone that plays a crucial role in sexual function. Inadequate sleep can lead to decreased testosterone levels, which may contribute to ED.

Blood flow: Adequate sleep supports healthy blood circulation. Poor sleep can affect blood flow throughout your body, including to the penis. Insufficient blood flow to the penis is a common cause of ED.

Psychological factors: Lack of sleep can lead to increased stress, anxiety, and mood disturbances. These psychological factors can contribute to sexual dysfunction, as they can interfere with sexual arousal and performance.

Fatigue: Chronic sleep deprivation can lead to physical and mental fatigue, reducing your overall energy and interest in sexual activity.

Sleep-related disorders: Conditions like sleep apnea, which disrupt sleep patterns and lead to oxygen deprivation, can negatively impact erectile function. Treating sleep disorders can improve sexual health.

To maintain good erectile health through quality sleep, consider the following tips:

Establish a regular sleep schedule and create a sleep-conducive environment, such as a dark and quiet room.

Manage stress: Practice stress-reduction techniques, such as mindfulness, meditation, or deep breathing exercises, to help relax your mind and improve sleep quality.

Limit caffeine and alcohol: Avoid consuming caffeine and alcohol close to bedtime, as they can disrupt sleep patterns.

Address sleep disorders: If you suspect you have a sleep

disorder like sleep apnea, consult a healthcare professional for evaluation and treatment.

Maintain a healthy lifestyle: Eat a balanced diet, stay hydrated, and avoid smoking and excessive alcohol consumption to support overall health, including erectile health.

If you experience persistent erectile dysfunction or believe your sleep issues are affecting your sexual health, it's essential to consult a healthcare provider. They can help determine the underlying causes and recommend appropriate treatment options, which may include lifestyle changes, therapy, or medications to address ED or sleep disorders.

Smoking and Alcohol: Their Impact on ED

Smoking and excessive alcohol consumption can both have

a negative impact on erectile dysfunction (ED). Understanding how these habits affect ED can help individuals make informed decisions about their health and lifestyle. Here's how smoking and alcohol can contribute to ED:

Reduced blood flow: Smoking damages blood vessels and reduces blood flow throughout the body, including to the penis. Adequate blood flow is essential for achieving and maintaining an erection.

Narrowed arteries: Smoking can lead to atherosclerosis (hardening and narrowing of the arteries) by causing the buildup of plaque in the arteries. This condition can limit blood flow to the penis, making it difficult to achieve and sustain an erection.

Decreased nitric oxide: Nitric oxide is a chemical that helps relax and dilate blood vessels, allowing for increased blood flow to the penis. Smoking reduces nitric oxide levels, which can impair erectile function.

Hormonal imbalances: Smoking can negatively affect hormone levels, including testosterone, which is essential for sexual desire and function.

Psychological factors: Smoking can contribute to stress, anxiety, and depression, all of which can be linked to ED.

Alcohol and ED:

Central nervous system depression: Alcohol is a depressant that can interfere with the central nervous system. In moderate to excessive quantities, it can impair sexual arousal and performance.

Hormone disruption: Alcohol can disrupt hormone production, including lowering testosterone levels, which can impact sexual function.

Performance anxiety: Alcohol can impair judgment and decision-making, leading to potential sexual performance anxiety, which can contribute to ED.

Dehydration: Excessive alcohol consumption can lead to dehydration, which can affect blood circulation and sexual performance.

It's important to note that the severity of the impact on ED varies from person to person and depends on the amount and duration of smoking or alcohol consumption. Reducing or quitting these habits can lead to improvements in erectile function over time.

If you are experiencing ED and are a smoker or have a history of excessive alcohol consumption, it's advisable to seek medical advice. Your healthcare provider can assess your situation and provide guidance on quitting smoking, reducing alcohol intake, and addressing any underlying health issues contributing to ED. They may also recommend treatments for ED, such as medications or therapy, to help improve your sexual function.

CHAPTER FIVE
Natural Therapies
Acupuncture and Erectile Dysfunction:

Acupuncture is a traditional Chinese medicine technique that involves the insertion of thin needles into specific points on the body to stimulate the flow of energy. While research on the effectiveness of acupuncture for erectile dysfunction (ED) is limited, some studies suggest that it may have a positive impact. Here's what you should know:

Potential Benefits: Acupuncture may help improve ED by promoting relaxation, reducing stress, and enhancing blood flow. Some practitioners believe that acupuncture can restore the body's energy balance, which could positively influence sexual function.

Scientific Evidence: While some small-scale studies have shown promising results, more high-quality research is needed to establish acupuncture as a reliable treatment for ED. The effect is individual dependent.

Safety: Acupuncture is generally considered safe when performed by a qualified practitioner. However, it's essential to consult with a healthcare provider before pursuing acupuncture as a treatment for ED.

Complementary Therapy: Acupuncture can be used in conjunction with other ED treatments, such as lifestyle modifications, medications, and psychotherapy, to achieve better results.

Yoga and Meditation:

Yoga and meditation are holistic practices that can contribute to overall well-being, reduce stress, and improve mental and physical health. While they may not be direct cures for ED, they can help address the underlying psychological factors contributing to sexual dysfunction:

Stress Reduction: Yoga and meditation promote relaxation and stress reduction, which can help alleviate performance anxiety and stress-related ED.

Improved Blood Flow: Some yoga poses may enhance blood circulation, which is vital for erectile function.

Mind-Body Connection: Both yoga and meditation foster a stronger mind-body connection, which can improve sexual awareness and confidence.

Emotional Health: These practices can help manage depression and anxiety, which are common factors associated with ED.

Alternative Therapies to Consider

In addition to acupuncture, yoga, and meditation, several

other alternative therapies and lifestyle modifications can be considered for managing ED naturally:

Herbal Supplements: Some herbal remedies, such as ginseng, L-arginine, and maca root, have been studied for their potential benefits in improving erectile function. Consult with a healthcare provider before using any supplements.

Diet and Nutrition: A healthy diet that includes whole foods, antioxidants, and nutrients can support overall health and sexual function. Nutrients like zinc, vitamin D, and omega-3 fatty acids may have a positive impact on ED.

Pelvic Floor Exercises: Pelvic floor exercises, such as Kegel exercises, can strengthen the muscles that control erections and ejaculation. They may be beneficial for some individuals with ED.

Acupressure: Similar to acupuncture, acupressure involves applying pressure to specific points on the body to promote energy flow. While research is limited, it's considered safe and may be worth exploring.

Stress Management Techniques: Various stress management methods, such as biofeedback, progressive muscle relaxation, and aromatherapy, can complement ED treatment by reducing anxiety and stress.

It is crucial to consult with a healthcare professional before trying any alternative therapies for ED. They can provide personalized guidance, ensure that these therapies are safe and appropriate for your specific situation, and help you create a comprehensive treatment plan that may include lifestyle changes, counseling, or medication as needed.

CHAPTER SIX
Communication and Relationships
The Role of Communication:

Effective communication is a fundamental component of a healthy and satisfying intimate relationship, especially when dealing with issues like erectile dysfunction (ED). Here's how communication plays a crucial role:

Open and Honest Dialogue: Openly discussing ED and its impact on your relationship is essential. Both partners should feel comfortable sharing their thoughts, concerns, and feelings.

Reducing Stigma: ED can be a sensitive topic. Effective communication can help reduce the stigma surrounding it, allowing both partners to feel more at ease discussing their experiences.

Understanding and Empathy: Communication fosters

understanding and empathy. It allows partners to comprehend each other's emotions and experiences, reducing frustration and resentment.

Mutual Support: Communicating about ED enables partners to support each other emotionally and provide reassurance. This mutual support can help strengthen the relationship.

Problem-Solving: Effective communication allows couples to work together to find solutions to ED-related issues. Discussing potential treatments, lifestyle changes, or counseling can lead to better outcomes.

Keeping the Spark Alive in Your Relationship

Maintaining a strong and passionate relationship while dealing with ED is essential. Below are some essential tips that can help to keep your spark alive:

Embrace Intimacy: Remember that intimacy goes beyond sexual intercourse. Emotional closeness, affection, and physical touch can keep your connection strong.

Try New Things: Explore new ways to connect and enjoy each other's company. This can include trying new hobbies, taking trips, or simply spending quality time together.

Focus on Emotional Connection: Build a strong emotional bond through regular communication, shared experiences, and being attentive to each other's needs.

Be Patient: Be patient with each other as you navigate the challenges of ED. Understand that setbacks may occur, but maintaining a positive attitude and supporting each other can make a difference.

Seek Professional Advice: Don't hesitate to consult with a healthcare provider or therapist for guidance on addressing

ED and its impact on your relationship.

Seeking Professional Help if Needed

When dealing with ED and its impact on your relationship, professional help can be beneficial in various ways:

Medical Evaluation: If you or your partner is experiencing ED, consult a healthcare provider for a thorough evaluation. They can identify any underlying physical or medical causes and recommend appropriate treatment options.

Counseling or Therapy: Couples counseling or sex therapy can be valuable for addressing relationship issues related to ED. A trained therapist can help improve communication, intimacy, and emotional connection.

Medication and Treatment Options: If the ED is primarily of a physical nature, your healthcare provider may prescribe medications or recommend other treatments to improve erectile function.

Support Groups: Consider joining a support group for individuals and couples dealing with ED. Sharing experiences and advice with others in a similar situation can provide comfort and valuable insights.

Education: Learn more about ED together. Understanding the condition and its potential causes can help both partners feel less anxious and more informed.

Remember that ED is a common issue, and it doesn't have to define your relationship. With open communication, mutual support, and professional guidance, you can overcome the challenges and maintain a satisfying and fulfilling relationship.

CHAPTER SEVEN
Case Studies and the Future of Natural Remedy
Real-Life Success Stories

In this chapter, we will explore real-life success stories of individuals and couples who faced and overcame erectile dysfunction (ED). These stories serve as inspiration and examples of how different people navigated the challenges of ED and found solutions to improve their sexual health and relationships. While each case is unique, common themes and lessons can be drawn from these experiences.

John and Sarah's Journey: John experienced ED due to stress and anxiety. They decided to seek couples counseling to address their communication issues and relationship stress. Through therapy and relaxation techniques, they improved their emotional connection, reduced stress, and rekindled their intimacy.

Mark's Lifestyle Changes: Mark, a smoker and heavy drinker, developed ED. He decided to quit smoking and limit alcohol consumption. Alongside a healthier diet and regular exercise, he saw a significant improvement in his erectile function.

Robert's Medical Treatment: Robert's ED was linked to a medical condition. After consulting a urologist, he was prescribed medication to improve his sexual function. The treatment was successful in helping him achieve and maintain erections.

Lessons and Inspiration from Others:

From these case studies, several valuable lessons and inspirations emerge:

Communication is Key: Open and honest communication with a partner is crucial for addressing ED and maintaining a healthy relationship. Seek professional help when necessary to facilitate these conversations.

Lifestyle Changes Matter: Lifestyle modifications, such as quitting smoking, reducing alcohol consumption, and adopting a healthier diet, can have a significant impact on erectile function.

Professional Guidance: Consulting healthcare providers and therapists can lead to effective treatment plans and improved emotional connection within a relationship.

Patience and Perseverance: Overcoming ED may require time and patience. Understand that progress can be gradual, but with a positive attitude and a commitment to seeking solutions, improvements are possible.

Holistic Approach: Addressing ED often requires a multifaceted approach that combines medical, psychological, and lifestyle interventions. Don't hesitate to explore different options and tailor your approach to your specific needs.

Sharing Stories: By sharing stories and experiences, individuals and couples facing ED can provide support and encouragement to others in similar situations. Learning from others' experiences can be a source of motivation.

These case studies demonstrate that ED is a treatable condition, and there is hope for improvement. By learning from the experiences of others, individuals and couples can find inspiration and guidance on their own journey toward better sexual health and fulfilling relationships. Remember that seeking professional help when needed is a valuable step in addressing ED effectively.

Ongoing Research and Developments:

As our understanding of erectile dysfunction (ED) and natural remedies continues to evolve, ongoing research and developments are shaping the future of ED treatments. Here are some areas of focus in current research:

Herbal Supplements: Scientists are conducting studies to further investigate the potential benefits of herbal supplements like ginseng, L-arginine, and maca root. Research aims to clarify their mechanisms of action and efficacy for improving erectile function.

Nutritional Interventions: Ongoing research explores the role of nutrition in ED. Scientists are studying specific diets, nutrients, and dietary patterns that may positively affect sexual health.

Exercise and Physical Activity: Research continues to emphasize the role of regular physical activity in maintaining erectile function. Studies aim to provide more insights into the type, intensity, and duration of exercises that have the greatest impact.

Psychological Interventions: Therapies such as mindfulness, meditation, and cognitive-behavioral techniques are under investigation for their potential to address psychological factors contributing to ED.

Biotechnological Innovations: Advances in biotechnology and regenerative medicine may lead to novel approaches for treating ED. Stem cell therapy and tissue engineering are areas of research that hold promise.

Promising Trends in Natural Erectile Dysfunction Treatments

While research is ongoing, several promising trends are emerging in the realm of natural remedies for ED:

Personalized Approaches: Tailoring treatments to an individual's unique needs and factors, such as lifestyle, genetics, and psychological profile, is gaining importance. Today, personalizing any treatment plans have become common and very popular.

Telemedicine and Digital Health: The use of telemedicine and digital health platforms is increasing, making it more convenient for individuals to access professional advice and resources for managing ED, including natural remedies.

Multidisciplinary Care: Combining various natural remedies, lifestyle changes, and psychological interventions in a comprehensive treatment plan is becoming a preferred approach. Healthcare providers are working collaboratively to address both physical and psychological aspects of ED.

Holistic Health Focus: Emphasizing overall health and well-being as a means to improve sexual health is gaining momentum. Natural remedies are often considered as part of a broader strategy for enhancing one's quality of life.

Non-Invasive Treatments: Many individuals prefer non-invasive or minimally invasive treatments for ED. Natural remedies align well with this preference, as they often involve lifestyle changes and supplements rather than surgical procedures or medications.

Research and Education: As our understanding of ED grows, education and awareness about the condition and its treatments are increasing. This will help you in making some well-informed decisions about your sexual health.

The future of natural remedies for ED looks promising, as ongoing research and developments continue to uncover new possibilities and refine existing approaches. With a growing focus on holistic health, personalized care, and multidisciplinary approaches, individuals dealing with ED can look forward to more effective and tailored solutions in the years to come. It is essential to consult with healthcare providers and stay informed about the latest advancements in the field.

Your Path to Natural Erectile Dysfunction Remedy

In this comprehensive guide, we have explored the various facets of natural remedies for erectile dysfunction (ED), providing you with valuable insights into the causes, lifestyle modifications, dietary changes, exercise, alternative therapies, and the role of communication in addressing ED naturally. Armed with this knowledge, you are well-equipped to embark on a journey to improve your sexual health using natural and holistic approaches.

The Journey Ahead

Dealing with ED is a journey that may require dedication, patience, and an openness to trying different methods. It's essential to remember that the path to improvement is unique to each individual. Seeking professional guidance when necessary is crucial, as healthcare providers can offer personalized advice and tailored treatment options based on your specific circumstances.

In conclusion, addressing ED with natural remedies is not only a viable approach but one that emphasizes overall health and well-being. By incorporating lifestyle changes, effective communication, and, when necessary, professional assistance, you can take significant steps toward enhancing your sexual health and improving your quality of life. You are not alone on this journey, and there is a wealth of support

and information available to assist you at every stage.

About the Book

In this guide, Mrs. Vera Jacob will journey you through:

Holistic approaches that have to do with, exploring the interconnectedness of physical, mental, and emotional well-being with ED.

Nutritional Insights helps to explore the impact of nutrition on erectile health and how to incorporate nutrient-rich foods and supplements that have the potency to support vascular health and improve blood flow.

Lifestyle Strategies that will explore lifestyle changes and the implementation of positive habits that contribute to increased vitality and sexual well-being.

Herbal Remedies includes the exploration of the world of herbal remedies known for their positive effects on male sexual health.

The Mind-Body Connection and empowerment of one to explore the connection between the mind and body in the realm of sexual health and to take charge of your sexual health in a supportive and informative manner.